HIGH BLOOD PRESSURE SOLUTION

HOW TO PREVENT AND TREAT HYPERTENTION, STROKE and CKD-With medication, Herbal, Essential Oils and Natural Remedies

By Beatrice Jonas

Copy right

This document is geared towards providing exact and reliable information in regards to the topic and issue covered. The publication is sold with the idea that the publisher is not required to render accounting, officially permitted, or otherwise, qualified services. If advice is necessary, legal or professional, a practiced individual in the profession should be ordered.

- From a Declaration of Principles which was accepted and approved equally by a Committee of the American Bar Association and a Committee of Publishers and Associations.

In no way is it legal to reproduce, duplicate, or transmit any part of this document in either electronic means or in printed format. Recording of this publication is strictly prohibited and any storage of this document is not allowed unless with written permission from the publisher. All rights reserved.

The information provided herein is stated to be truthful and consistent, in that any liability, in terms of inattention or otherwise, by any usage or abuse of any policies, processes, or directions

TABLE OF CONTENT

CHAPTER ONE

HIGH BLOOD PRESSURE

According to the American Heart Association, "Blood pressure measure the force exerted by blood pushing outwards on your arteries walls" .The amount of force, exerted against the walls of the arteries is known as high blood. High blood pressure can also be commonly referred to as Hypertension. Studies have shown that about 72million people in the USA have high blood pressure. The National Heart Lung and Blood institute state that one out of three adults *has High Blood Pressure. While the National institute of Health (NIH) states that almost 2\3 (two thirds) of people above the age of 65 in the United States of America have high blood pressure.*

The National Health Service in the United Kingdom (UK) states that about 40% of adults in Britain have high blood pressure. Also, there are reports that high blood pressure (HBP) is more common amongst people of the African origin in the USA than the Caucasians. Men tend to have high blood pressure (HBP) than women before the age of 45. From age 45-54, both men and women seem to have same blood pressure (BP).

This observation is really shocking. But what is more shocking is the fact that when you compare the lifestyle of men and women of this age group, men are more involved in the things that can contribute to high blood pressure and Stroke. Men of this age - drink more, smoke more and see their doctor less- maybe just to avoid confessing their sins of alcohol and cigarette smoking to doctors. Yet, over 55,000 more women suffer Hypertension and Stroke than men every year. But from age 55-64 and above, women tend to have high blood pressure (HBP) than men. In general, anyone who has a high blood pressure of 140/90 mmHg and above for a set period of time is said to have high blood pressure (HBP).

If your doctor or health care provider measures your blood pressure and states that it reads 120/80 mmHg, it means that your systolic (top) reading is 120 mmHg while your diastolic (bottom) is 80 mmHg. The term SYSTOLIC & DIASTOLIC pressure represents the blood pressure readings when the heart is contracting and when the heart is resting or expanding.

Note: mmHg means - millimeter Mercury.

STAGES OF HIGH BLOOD PRESSURE (H.B.P)

There are different stages of high blood pressure or Hypertension, they are;

1) Normal blood pressure: when your blood pressure reading is less than 120/80 mmHg, it is referred to as normal blood pressure.

2) Pre-hypertension: when your blood pressure reading is between 120-139 over 80-89 (mmHg), the condition is referred to as Pre-hypertension.

3) Stage 1 high blood pressure (HBP): any blood pressure reading that is between 140-159mmHg over 90-99mmHg is known as stage 1 HBP.

4) Stage two (II) high blood pressure: blood pressure reading of 160mmHg and above over 100mmHg and above is known as stage 2 HBP.

Note: People of age 60 years and above mostly have blood pressure reading of 150/90 mmHg and above.

TYPES OF HIGH BLOOD PRESSURE (HYPERTENSION)

There are two major types of hypertension, they are:

1) Primary/Essential hypertension: In this type, the main cause of hypertension is not yet known. Although, it has been traced to some risk factors which may include: family history, gender, age, race, lifestyle, diet, stress, obesity, diabetes, lack of magnesium, potassium, calcium, excessive consumption

of alcohol, lack of physical exercise and other social and environmental factors.

2) Secondary hypertension: when the main cause of high blood pressure is identifiable, it is known as secondary hypertension. In this case, your doctor or healthcare provider may need to treat the underlying cause(s) such as disease and other ailments.

Among the other prevailing known cause of secondary hypertension, kidney disease ranks most. Also, tumors, pregnancy, birth control pills and medications that narrow blood vessels can increase blood pressure.

SIGNS AND SYMPTOMS OF

HYPERTENSION (HBP)

As the primary underlying cause of high blood pressure is not known, its signs and symptoms can remain undetected for a long period of time. This is why hypertension is often referred to as "silent killer". It is actually possible for someone to be hypertensive without knowing about it. Hence, it is recommended that you check your blood pressure regularly/occasionally either with sphygmomanometers from your health care provider or Fitbit, an instrument you can wear around your wrist to determine your blood pressure.

The symptoms of high blood pressure usually begin after chronic hypertension, a condition in which the blood pressure reading is about 180/110 mmHg and above.

The symptoms include the following:

1) Fatigue

2) Headache

3) Dizziness

4) Blurred vision

5) Dyspnea (shortness of breath or breathlessness)

Complicated signs and symptoms of high blood pressure may include the following:

1) Stroke: A condition in which blood flow to the brain is partially blocked (partial stroke) or permanently blocked (severe stroke). The symptoms of stroke includes: paralysis of the legs, arms, inability to speak or understand speech etc.

2) Heart failure: A condition in which the heart pumps insufficient blood to meet the required blood supply needed by the body. Symptoms may include: swelling in the

abdomen, ankles, legs, feet, difficulty in breathing etc.

3) Chronic kidney disease (CDK): This condition may occur when the blood vessels constricts in the kidney thereby leading to kidney failure.

4) Partial blindness: This condition occurs when there is bleeding in the blood vessels connected to the eyes.

5) Brain rupture: This condition is mainly associated with the secondary hypertension. Blood clots around the wall of the brain, thereby causing blockage to blood flow in the brain cell. It takes several conditions and

proper treatments for patient to recover from this type of condition.

6) Heart attack: This occurs, when the oxygen needed by the heart is suddenly blocked and the oxygen rich blood needed by the parts of the heart muscles become restricted. It may results to the following; shortness of breath, chest pain and discomfort in the upper body.

7) Cognitive changes: This condition may results due to higher number of blood pressure, for example, values higher than 189/110 mmHg. It symptoms include; loss of focus during conversation, memory loss, difficulties in making speech etc.

CHAPTER TWO

MEASUREMENT OF BLOOD

PRESSURE

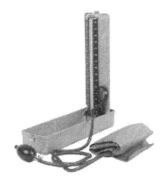

Sphygmomanometer

The instrument that is mainly used by healthcare providers to measure blood pressure reading is called sphygmomanometer. Its function is science based. It's also able to determine ones blood pressure when inserted into the right position. You can also determine your blood pressure by using Fitbit, an instrument that can be tied to the wrist like a hand band or wristwatch to determine your blood pressure readings.

HOW TO RECORD BLOOD PRESSURE READING

A single blood pressure reading is not enough to determine whether someone is hypertensive or not. Hence, you may need to take several readings at different times, conditions and locations to know your actual blood pressure readings.

Sometimes, your personal blood pressure readings may be different from your doctor's reading. It's not because you were wrong or your instrument malfunctioned. No, it may simply be, because you were anxious or stressed during your visit to your doctor or maybe you ate not long before visiting your doctor, many factors could be responsible.

When taking blood pressure readings either at home or in the office by yourself for the first time, it's important for you to know that there is variation between the left arm and the right arm blood pressure readings. The variation between the right arm and the left arm should be 10mmHg or less. Any value higher than 10mmHg is abnormal and should be discussed with your healthcare provider (National Institute of Health).

If you are measuring your blood pressure for the very first time, either in your doctor's office or at home, it is recommended that you take the readings in both arms. If one arm continually has higher blood pressure reading than the other, that arm should be used to take your blood pressure readings.

I have personally had experiences in which the values of my blood pressure readings taken in my doctor's office goes high compared to the values obtained in other locations. I discussed this condition with my doctor and he said it is sometimes normal with patients. He said the condition is known as *"white coat hypertension"* and could be as a result of stress, anxiety, anxiousness etc.

Therefore, *"white coat hypertension"* is a condition in which the readings of your blood pressure are only high when measured in the office of your healthcare provider compared to readings obtained in other places.

As stated earlier, the top values in your blood pressure readings is known as systolic (less than 120mmHg for normal blood pressure) while the bottom value is known as diastolic (usually less than 80mmHg for normal blood pressure).

LIST OF THINGS TO AVOID BEFORE MEASURING BLOOD PRESSURE

1) Do not smoke or drink alcohol or caffeinated drink before/during measuring blood pressure.

2) Do not eat anything within 30 minutes before taking your blood pressure reading.

3) Do not engage in any form of exercise within 30 minutes before taking your blood pressure readings.

4) Do not conclude the final result of your blood pressure reading on just one or two readings taken in a minute apart.

5) Do not take readings at different times of the day. Make sure that your blood pressure readings are taken at almost exactly the same time each day either in the morning before breakfast or in the evening.

CHAPTER THREE

HOW TO PREVENT

HYPERTENSION, STROKE AND

CKD

The best way to prevent high blood pressure is to maintain a healthy lifestyle habit which may include: physical exercises for your body, eating healthy meals, avoid excessive consumption of alcohol, maintain healthy body weight, quit smoking, drink plenty of water, and get enough of sleep (7-8 hours daily) etc.

If you have been diagnosed of pre-hypertension, it is important to check your blood pressure regularly and discuss with your healthcare provider. Also, you may need to change your lifestyle habit and follow prescribed recommendations and treatment plans by your healthcare provider. A healthy lifestyle can reverse the condition of pre-hypertension, prevents complications, helps to control existing hypertension and helps to curb long term problems of high blood pressure such as stroke, heart failure, chronic kidney disease (CKD), heart attack etc.

HOW TO PREVENT STROKE

There is a strong connection between high blood pressure (HBP) and stroke. In fact, stroke is the end point of untreated high blood pressure. According to Dr. Rost *"High blood pressure is the biggest contributor to the risk of stroke in both men and women"*

Funny enough, over 20 percent of the people living with high blood pressure are unaware of their condition. Hence, these classes of people are more susceptible to having stroke.

Some people, especially those of the African origin had linked stroke to spiritualism – saying, it is a sickness from the spirit world or from their ancestors. This type of belief has no evidence. Others say, it is genetic – which mean, either they inherited it or it can be inherited due to long family history. This might be true, as evidence had shown connection between family history and their blood pressure in many cases. Despite this belief, with the right method and treatment, stroke can be managed.

Here are some ways to prevent stroke

(1) If you have been diagnosed of stage 1 or stage 2 hypertension ($^{140}/_{90}mmHg$ and above, $^{160}/_{110}\ mmHg\ and\ above$) then you will need to monitor your heartbeat by checking it regularly at least once in a month by your healthcare provider.

(2) Treat diabetes: Having high blood sugar can damage blood vessels which might lead to blood clotting in the blood vessels thereby resulting in partial or severe stroke.

Hence, there is need to monitor and keep your blood sugar level normal.

(3) If you are overweight or suffer from obesity, losing as little as 10 pounds weight will do much to help reduce your chances of having stroke.

(4) Use exercise: Just as little exercise of 30 – 45 minutes can help in regulating blood pressure; it can also help to reduce the chances of having stroke. Therefore, exercise at least 30 – 45 minutes in 5days a week, Follow our exercise plan.

(5) If you are an addicted smoker and drunkard, quit both or reduce smoking and drinking of alcohol to it minimum level.

(6) Learn to sleep for at least 7 hours per night and avoid social activities that might increase your chances of having stroke once you have been diagnosed of stage 1 or stage II hypertension. − Activities like staying awake in the night for clubbing, gamming and from poker house.

(7) Use essential oils: Make olive oil your essential cooking oil. It has the chance of reducing stroke by 40%.

(8) When you suffer from continuous migraine, it can increase your chances of having high blood pressure (HBP) and stroke. Please discuss with your healthcare provider for the right treatment.

(9) Eat sweet potatoes, banana, raisins, and tomatoes because they have high level of potassium which can help to lower the risk of having high blood pressure and stroke by 20%.

SIGNS and SYMPTONS

See the table below for explanation

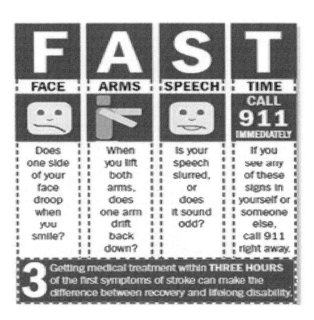

HOW TO PREVENT CHRONIC KIDNEY DISEASE (CKD)

The American Kidney Fund states that "*An estimated 31 million people in the united states are living with Chronic Kidney Disease (CKD)*". Even with this alarming figure, many people do not take their health issues serious, especially those, that are hypertensive, and are addicted to drinking excess alcohol and smoking cigarettes.

Some common factors that can increase your chances of having stroke are:

1. High blood pressure (HBP)

2. Diabetes

3. Family and genetic factor

4. Heart disease

5. Age. 60 years and above

6. Race. African – Americans have high risk than Caucasians.

Symptoms of Chronic Kidney Disease (CKD)

1. Swelling in your ankles and feet.

2. Passing of excess urine

3. Shortness in breath or difficulty in breathing

4. Sleeplessness

5. Muscle cramps etc.

Complicated kidney disease symptoms may include:

1. Diarrhea

2. Vomiting

3. Back pain

4. Bleeding from the nose

5. Abdominal pain

6. Anemia

7. Heart disease

8. Heart failure.

HOW TO PREVENT STROKE

There is a strong link between high blood pressure, diabetes and stroke. If you have been diagnosed of hypertension or diabetes, it is important that you work with your health care provider to work on lowering your blood pressure and keeping your blood sugar level under control.

Here are some things to practice:

1. Cut your salt and sodium intake to the daily recommended values

2.   Exercise

3.   Quick smoking and drinking of alcohol when you are hypertensive.

Unfortunately, there is no cure treatment for damaged kidney. One may need a kidney transplant once the kidney is labeled damaged.

CHAPTER FOUR

HOW TO TREAT HIGH BLOOD

PRESSURE

There are different methods of treating high blood pressure or hypertension. For the purpose of this book, we are going to briefly discuss how to treat hypertension (HBP) with the followings:

1) *Medication (medicine)*

2) Essential oils

3) Herbal and supplements

4) Natural remedies

Medications (medicine) For Treating Hypertension or HBP

Although this is not a medical textbook, it will make a common sense to suggest drugs that can help in treating high blood pressure. Note that the information contained here is never intended to replace your healthcare provider recommendations and suggestions. Make sure you discuss with your doctor before using any of these drugs;

1) **Thiazide diuretics**: This drug can help to eliminate sodium and water from our body by acting on the kidney.

2) **Angiotensin Converting Enzyme (ACE) inhibitors**: It helps to reduce blood pressure by blocking some hormones in our body system.

3) **Calcium channel blockers**: This drug helps to regulate blood pressure by decreasing the amount of calcium in the blood vessels.

4) **Beta blockers**: This drug has the ability to slow down heart rate and also to reduce the force of the heart thereby lowering blood pressure.

Complicated cases of hypertension or high blood pressure (HBP) may include the use of the following medicines:

1) Alpha-beta blockers

2) Central-acting agents

3) Alpha blockers

Note: all drugs mentioned here have different potential side effects; they should be taken based on recommendation by healthcare providers.

HERBAL AND SUPPLEMENTS TREATMENTS FOR HIGH BLOOD PRESSURE

If you are currently on any treatment plan due to hypertension or you are a stage 1 or stage 2 high blood pressure sufferers, it is recommended that you discuss with your healthcare provider before turning to herbal treatments.

1) **Cardamom**: This herb is used in the food of south Asians especially in India. Studies revealed that it has the ability to reduce high blood pressure. It can be used as spice in powder form for soup and stew.

2) **Basil**: Extracts from basil had been known to reduce blood pressure. Fresh basil can be directly added to our diets to enjoy the benefits of the delicious herb.

3) **Cinnamon**: Daily consumption of cinnamon has been revealed to lower blood pressure for diabetic patients. It can be

sprinkled directly on our breakfast to improve the flavor of stew, curries and stir-fries.

4) **Garlic**: Although Garlic has offensive odor and the ability to ruin one's breath, it is believed to have the capacity to lower blood pressure by making the blood vessels dilate and relax. Garlic can be added to your favorite recipe list if you fancy it but if you think the offensive odor of garlic is too strong for you, then, you can roast it before use or take it as supplement.

5) **Flax seed**: Flaxseeds contain omega-3 fatty acids which can significantly lower

blood pressure. Flaxseed can also be used as anti-oxidant and helps to protect against cardiovascular disease by reducing cholesterol. Flax seed can be bought grounded or you can grind it yourself using coffee grinder. It can virtually be added to any dish.

6) **Celery seed**: This herb is used to cure hypertension in china. You can either use the seed or juice the entire plant to lower blood pressure. It has been found to be Diuretic which might make it to be effective in lowering blood pressure. Celery seed can

be used to flavor casseroles, stews, soups and other delicious dishes.

7) **Ginger**: It has the ability to enhance blood circulation and rest the muscles surrounding blood vessel. It is almost used globally as vegetable dishes, soups or ingredient for beverages.

8) **Cat's claw**: It is used in china by traditional health practitioners to treat neurological health problems and hypertension. It contains calcium which might be responsible for its effectiveness in

reducing blood pressure. It is readily available as supplement in many health food stores.

9) **Hawthorn**: This herb had been used for years in the Chinese traditional medicine to reduce high blood pressure. Hawthorn has the ability to prevent clot formation, reduce blood pressure and improve blood circulation. It can be taken as a tea, pill or liquid extract.

10. **French Lavender**: Lavender oil is mainly used for perfuming and

cosmetic products. Yet this herb has the power to lower blood pressure. Lavender leaves can be used just the same way Rosemary leaf is used.

In conclusion, if you are a stage 1 or stage 2 blood pressure sufferers, it is highly advisable that you check your blood pressure regularly, and also discuss with your doctor before using any herbal medicine.

ESSENTIAL OILS FOR HIGH BLOOD PRESSURE TREATMENT

Essential oils have the power to lower blood pressure by dilating arteries, reducing emotional stress and playing the role of anti-oxidant. Although essential oils can lower blood pressure, but not all essential oils are safe for this purpose.

Some safe essential oils include; Frankincense, Ylang-ylang, Lavender, Marjoram, Cypress, Bergamot and Clary

FRANKINCENSE OIL

Frankincense oil has the power to reduce stress, anxiety and anger. It also promotes relaxation and good breathing. Due to it sedative nature, it has the ability to restore mental state to calmness. Add some drops of frankincense oil to a diffuser or vaporizer to manage stress and lower high blood pressure.

You can make a blend of essential oil by incorporating the following essential oils;

Half (1/2) ounce Simple Salve

15 drops of Ylang-ylang

7 drops of frankincense oil

7 drops of Cypress

7 drops of Marjoram oil.

PROCEDURE

Mix all the essential oils together in a clean bowl, stir using a toothpick or small stick, and allow the mixture to settle overnight. Rub the blend around your chest area twice daily (morning and evening) for quick and effective results.

YLANG-YLANG OIL

Ylang-ylang oil contains a sweet aroma that is highly effective in clearing nervous tension, stress, agitation and also promotes good sleep.

LAVENDER OIL

Lavender oil has the ability to balance emotion, relief stress and helps to soothe the body. The incredible sweet aroma of lavender oil can be used to treat depression, nervous disorder and unbalanced emotions. Due to its relaxing property, it is able to calm nervous system and lower high blood pressure.

You can make a blend of essential oil as follows;

2 drops of Lavender oil

2 drops of Ylang-ylang oil

2 drops of Bergamot oil

15ml of Sweet Almond oil (serves as the carrier oil)

PROCEDURE

Mix all the oils in a clean bowl to make a powerful and effective blend of essential oil. Apply on the body after bath in the evening while giving attention to the chest area. This blend can be used to massage the body to relief stress, lower high blood pressure and for the treatment of stroke.

CLARY SAGE OIL

6 drops of Clary sage oil

6 drops of Marjoram oil

6 drops of Ylang-ylang oil

6 drops of Lavender oil.

PROCEDURE

Mix all the oils in a clean bowl. Apply on the body after bath in the evening while giving attention to the chest area.

CANOLA ESSENTIAL OILS

According to Health Research and Toxicology, Research Division in Ottawa Canada, Canola essential oils is not regarded as a safe essential oil due to many factors which includes the following effects; heart problems, poor memory, dry skin, autoimmune disease, kidney disease, liver malfunction, high risk of cancer amongst other health challenges.

One (1) cup of canola oil has the following nutritional value. Hence, it safety for human consumption is subject to doubt.

Saturated fat (16g-80% RDV)

Calories 1927

Total fat 218g-335 RDV

Vitamin K (155mg-194% RDV), Vitamin E (38.1mg-190%)

Trans fat- 1g

RDV- Recommended Daily Value.

The irony of canola oil for the treatment of high blood pressure is that it actually increases high blood pressure, introduces oxidized cholesterol which can lead to cardiovascular disease and high risk of cancer. Therefore, canola oil is not regarded safe for human consumption. Canola oil should be replaced with coconut oil which is very safe both for cooking and otherwise.

NATURAL REMEDIES FOR HYPERTENSION

Well-tailored natural methods for treating high blood pressure will comprise the followings:

A) Healthy lifestyle.

B) The use of natural food or diet to lower or control high blood pressure.

C) The use of physical exercises to keep our body active.

TOP FOODS FOR BLOOD PRESSURE CONTROL

1) **Omega-3 rich foods**: Foods like Chia seeds, flax seeds, grass fed beef, and wild salmon can reduce inflammation.

2) **High potassium foods**: banana, melons and avocados are high in potassium, which can help to eliminate the effects of sodium in our body.

3) **High fiber foods**: such as fruits and vegetables.

4) **Dark chocolates**: dark chocolate that contains about 200mg and above of cocoa phenols can help reduce blood pressure.

5) **Low sodium foods**.

CHAPTER FIVE

NATURAL REMEDY TIPS TO

LOWER BLOOD PRESSURE

The practice of the following tips could make the difference between the old you and the new you. Use these five (5) secret methods to rejuvenate your body system, make your heart stronger and resurrect the dead cells in your body. Now, you can have the inner strength to act younger and be more energetic just like an 18 years old child. (wink)

A) Daily consumption of 1000-2000mg of fish oil can help to reduce inflammation and reduce blood pressure when taken for a long period of time.

B) Consumption of recommended dose of potassium supplements by your healthcare provider can help to lower your high blood pressure.

C) Consumption of about 600mg of garlic extracts can help to relax our muscles and also lower blood pressure.

D) Taking 500mg of magnesium supplement before going to bed can help to relax our muscles and also to reduce blood pressure.

FOODS THAT CAN LOWER BLOOD PRESSURE

The importance of the nutrients contained in these foods listed below cannot be over emphasized. Hence it is good that you add them to your meal plans. As intended, this is not a recipe book that teaches on how to prepare foods, rather it is a guide that shows list of foods that can possibly help to reduce hypertension together with the ways to cope, manage and overcome the problems associated with high blood pressure, Stroke and chronic kidney disease (CKD)

Potatoes, peas, celery, papaya, green beans, guava, oat meal, tomatoes, plain yoghurt, kiwis, blueberries, avocadoes, spinach, prunes, cantaloupe, dandelion, carrots, salmon, skim milk, beets, water, oranges, banana, raisins, sunflower seeds, tilapia, pork tenderloin (for meat lowers, it contains 6% of magnesium and 15% of potassium), peaches and Nectarines.

LIST OF FOODS TO AVOID

Below are the lists of foods that can increase blood pressure:

Processed deli meat, frozen pizza, salt and sodium (1,500mg or lower daily), canned soup, pickles, refined sugar, coffee, alcohol, package foods and chicken skin, caffeine, fast foods. Your goal should be 5-9 servings of fruits and vegetables.

In conclusion, the natural remedies for high blood pressure are:

1) Sip some hibiscus.

2) Reduce the intake of salt and sodium.

3) Drink fish oil according to the volume indicated at the bottle label.

4) Drink coconut water.

5) Eat hawthorn.

6) Eat watermelon especially in the morning.

7) Drink ginger tea.

8) Use garlic in your food.

9) Drink cat's claw concoction.

10) Eat blueberry.

11) Exercise your body.

CHAPTER SIX

THE EFFECT OF SALT IN OUR BODY

Salt in the kidney can make the body to retain excess water. This excessive water storage due to high level of salt can raise the body blood pressure and limit the function of the brain, kidney, heart and the arteries.

EFFECTS AND FUNCTIONS OF SODIUM IN OUR BODY

Honestly, sodium is not a bad mineral in our body; it is regarded as an essential mineral needed by our body. It helps to control the fluid balance in our body and functions to send nerve impulses and affect the way our muscles function. But excess consumption of sodium beyond the daily recommended level can pose some health risk to our body. The daily recommended consumption of sodium is 1,500mg, but when our body contains high level of sodium beyond the recommended level, it tends to pull water into our blood vessels thereby increasing the level of blood flowing in the blood vessels and then increases our blood pressure - According to INTERSALT study (adapted from INTERSALT study, 1988).

Several studies have shown that salt is mainly responsible for high blood pressure condition in the united states of America (USA) and the united kingdom (UK) than any other contributing factors such as; consumption of dairy foods, low in-take of potassium, excess consumption of alcohol, obesity and lack of physical exercises. (The U.S centers for disease control and prevention (CDC) 2009).

DIFFERENCES BETWEEN SALT

AND SODIUM

Common salt or table salt is a combination of two minerals, sodium and chloride. The sodium content is about 60%. Approximately 90% of Americans sodium intake in-take is from sodium chloride. Also, about 77% of sodium we consume comes from processed and refined foods. People that have been diagnosed of stage 1 and stage II hypertension should limit their salt consumption to maximum of 6g per day according to the UK National Health Service.

SOME COMMON FOODS THAT ARE HIGH IN SODIUM

1. Canned soup.

2. Deli meat.

3. Processed foods such as sausage, ham, bacon, lunch meat, Frozen and boxed mixes for rice, pasta and potatoes.

4. Others include; fast food snacks (peanuts, popcorn, chips) marinated food, regular salad dressing, butter and margarine.

The three key minerals that can help to control high blood pressure are;

a) Potassium.

b) Calcium.

c) Magnesium.

POTASSIUM

Potassium has the ability to counter the effect of sodium in our body system. The daily recommended dose of potassium for an adult is about 4,700mg. According to the Dietary Approaches to Stop Hypertension (D.A.S.H), common foods that are rich in vegetables, fruits, whole grains, low fat, beans, fish, and unsalted nuts are found to be effective in reducing systolic and diastolic blood pressure by about 5.5/3.0mmHg compared to other foods that are commonly consumed by about 75% of Americans that contains more than the recommended level of salt and sodium.

Potassium is an important nutrient needed by the body for the maintenance of fluid and electrolyte balance in the body. Potassium deficiency can cause the following health problems; Hypertension, irritability and fatigue. It is always impossible to have overdose of potassium, except through consumption of potassium salt, which may cause cardiac arrest, Nausa and vomiting.

Here are some common foods that have high potassium nutrients;

S/N	Food & type	Potassium content (mg)	Serving size (g)	Daily value (%)
1	Dried Apricots	1162	100	33
2	White Beans	561	100	16
3	Baked Acorn squash	437	100	12
4	Dark leafy greens (spinach):	558	100	16
5	Salmon fish:	628	100	18
6	White Mushrooms	396	100	11
7	Banana	358	100	10
8	Plain Yoghurt:	255	100	7
9	Baked Potassium:	535	100	15
10	Avocados:	485	100	14

FRUIT SOURCE OF POTASSIUM

INCLUDES:

S/N	Food & type	Potassium content (mg)	Serving size (g)	Daily value (%)
1	Passion fruit	348	100	10
2	Honeydew melon	228	100	7
3	Blackberries	162	100	5
4	Strawberries	153	100	4
5	Mangoes	168	100	5
6	Oranges	181	100	5
7	Grapes	191	100	5
8	Cherries	222	100	6
9	Watermelon	112	100	3
10	Apples	120	100	3

Vegetable Sources of Potassium

S/N	Food & type	Potassium content (mg)	Serving size (g)	Daily value (%)
1	Brussels sprout	398	100	11
2	Kale	491	100	14
3	Beet Greens	909	100	26
4	Garden Cress	606	100	17
5	Broccoli	343	100	10
6	Carrots	320	100	9
7	Cauliflower	299	100	9
8	Cooked Celery	284	100	8
9	Endive	314	100	9

MAGNESIUM

The recommended dose for magnesium depends on certain factors such as gender and age. Men between the ages of 19-30 years and above should have a daily intake of 400mg of magnesium. Men at the age of 31 years and above should have a daily intake of 420mg of magnesium.

For women between the ages of 19-30 years should have a daily intake of 310mg of magnesium while those at 31 years old and above should have a daily intake of 320mg of magnesium.

Magnesium: Our body needs magnesium to maintain normal muscle, keep the heartbeat normal, keep our immune system healthy, help build a stronger bone, and maintain nerve function.

When our body suffers from magnesium deficiency, we may experience the followings; Cerebral infraction, high blood pressure, diabetes, muscle spasms, cardiovascular disease, anxiety among others.

Just in the same way, that magnesium deficiency can have same adverse effect on our body, surplus or excess magnesium in our body may lead to diarrhea.

The table below shows some common foods that are rich in magnesium (100g)

S/N	Food & type	Mg content (mg)	Serving size (g)	Daily value (%)
1	Nuts and seeds	534	100	134
2	Soya beans	86	100	22
3	Mackerel fish	97	100	24
4	Brown rice	44	100	11
5	Dark chocolate	327	100	82
6	Plain yogurt	19	100	5

CALCIUM

People with high intake of calcium tend to have a stable or normal blood pressure. The recommended daily intake of calcium for adults between the ages of 19-50 years is 1,000mg while people above the age of 50 years should have a daily intake of 1,200mg of calcium.

Calcium had been proven to be safe and good for pregnant women and breastfeeding moms.

Calcium is an essential nutrient required by the body for growth and maintenance of strong bones, teeth, and for the secretion of enzymes and hormones. Calcium deficiency can lead to; Muscle cramps, abnormal breathing, convulsion, appetite loss amongst others.

Excess calcium in the body which may results intake of supplements can cause certain health challenges like; stroke, heart attack, kidney stone, etc.

The table below shows lists of foods and their calcium *Nutrients/contents in 100g.*

S/N	Food & type	Calcium Content (mg)	Serving Size (g)	Daily Value (%)
1	Tofu	350	100	35
2	Almond	264	100	26
3	Broccoli	47	100	5
4	Cooked Okra	77	100	8

5	Chinese Cabbage	105	100	11
6	Low Fat Yoghurt	183	100	18
7	Low fat Chesse	961	100	95

Vegetables High in calcium

S/N	Food type	Calcium contents (mg)	Serving size (g)	Daily value (DV) %
1	Arugula	160	100	16
2	Spring onions	72	100	7
3	Swiss chard	58	100	6
4	Leeks	59	100	6
5	Fennel	49	100	5
6	Rutabagas	43	100	4
7	Butternut squash	48	100	5

Fruits high in calcium

Name	Calcium Continent (mg)	Serving size (g)	Daily value (%)
Kumquats	62	100	6
Figs	35	100	4
Blackcurrants	55	100	6
Clementine	30	100	3
Lime	33	100	3
Kiwi fruit	34	100	4
Orange	40	100	4
Persimmons	27	100	3
Tangerines	37	100	4

CHAPTER SEVEN

HOW TO USE EXERCISE AND DIET TO LOWER HIGH BLOOD PRESSURE

Have you ever heard the saying? *"Even a little exercise profits the body"*. As we grow older, the chances of having high blood pressure increases. Hence, even the slightest form of exercise can be of immense benefit to our body. You don't need a rigorous exercise to control or lower your blood pressure, you might also not need to join a gym or run 100 meters race like Usain Bolt before you can lower your blood pressure. All you need is just to exercise your body for as little as 30-45 minutes, 5 days a week to have your desired results as a beginner.

RELATIONSHIP BETWEEN EXERCISE AND HIGH BLOOD PRESSURE (HYPERTENSION)

Research has shown that exercising our body regularly can make our hearts stronger- a condition that is good for the heart and blood pressure control. When the heart is strong enough, it pumps blood with little effort. Your being active in exercises has the potential to lower your systolic blood pressure by 4-9mmHg. To achieve your desired goal and to maintain a normal blood pressure of 120/80mmHg without depending on drugs and medicine, you need to carry out physical exercises for a long period of time.

The only flaw in the method is that your blood pressure may automatically increase as soon as you become inactive in physical exercises but who would want to change his winning team? I guess it is common sense to hold on to what is working. For me personally, I have decided to avoid the pains of swallowing pills and medicine just to control my blood pressure by using exercises to keep my body and heart fit and strong. The department of Health and Human Services recommends that adding strength-training exercise of all major muscle groups into a fitness routine at least twice a week.

HOW LONG DO I NEED TO EXERCISE MY BODY?

The Department of Health and Human Services recommends moderate aerobic activity for at least 150 minutes and 75 minutes of vigorous exercises in a week. Hence, you may need just about 30 minutes of aerobic exercises per day to keep your body and heart physically strong.

Some aerobic exercise may include; jogging, dancing, and rock climbing, climbing stairs, walking, bike riding etc. Weight training might also be an important exercise to help lower your blood pressure if you have stage 1 or stage II hypertension. To enjoy the benefits of physical exercise program and reduce the risk of injuries during exercise, you may need to start slowly. Warm up for at least 5 minutes before embarking on any of the exercises and also remember to rest afterward especially when you feel tired.

If you notice any strange occurrence during the period of exercising, discuss it immediately with your healthcare provider. Also, there is need to consult your healthcare provider before you begin any exercise plan so that he/she can help you select the one that best suits your situation. Some of the common signs you might experience when you first begin your exercise program include; jaw pain, chest pain, general body weakness, dizziness, shortage of breath, irregular heart beat etc.

SIMPLE EXERCISE PLAN FOR

BEGINNERS

Days	Exercise type	Time
Monday	Jogging/swimming	30-45 minutes
Tuesday	Dancing/walking	30-45 minutes
Wednesday	Rest	---
Thursday	Running/stairs climbing	30-45 minutes
Friday	Weight lifting	30-45 minutes
Saturday	Rock climbing/biking	30-45 minutes

You can interchange the exercise to choose the one that best suits your mood but make sure you are committed and dedicated to whatever plan you have adopted. When you have witnessed improvement in your health and blood pressure, you can increase the time required to complete each exercise for maximum benefit.

CONCLUSION

Despite the alarming figures and analysis from different reports, Hypertension, Stroke and Chronic Kidney Disease (CKD) can either be prevented or treated. We have tried our best to explain the different methods and types of treatment available—medication, herbal, essential oils and natural remedies through diet, lifestyle change and exercise.

When you combine the information contained in this books with your Doctor's advice and medication, you are guaranteed to overcome this sickness labeled ``Number one silent killer``.

In summary, you need - healthy lifestyle, Rest (7 hours of sleep at night), eat quality foods that are rich in Potassium, Calcium & Magnesium. Exercise for at least 30---45 minutes per day in 5 days a week, quit smoking and drinking of alcohol if you are hypertensive.

The best way to reward an author is to write a review. Kindly write your review on amazon.com, through the purchase link if you've enjoyed reading this book.

Once again, thanks for downloading and reading this book, I await your earnest review. See you there!

Beatrice Jonas

You can connect with us on our Facebook fan page @www.brainlisa@wealthcreator.com.

Made in the USA
San Bernardino, CA
13 October 2017